The Awesome Comp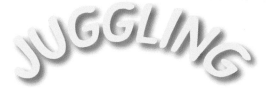

By Mike Murphy and Andy Murphy

AWESOME
Companion Books

a division of

Retro Ranger
Publishing Company

retrorangerpub.com

Awesome Companion Books
a division of
Retro Ranger Publishing Company,
Oshkosh, WI.

"To my dad
For teaching me a skill I can pass
on to my child and share as a
family tradition."

- *Andy Murphy*

"To my wife and family
You've encouraged me and
supported me through some
trying times and I can't thank you
enough."

"Juggling taught me that with
time and perseverance you can
accomplish almost anything."

- *Mike Murphy*

What is an Awesome Companion Book?

The Awesome Companion Books are a series of 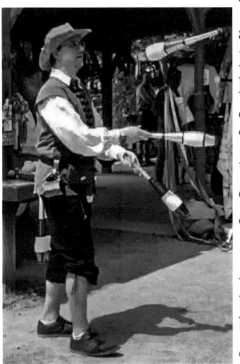 "How To" guides for adults and children. Each book in the series has a companion book designed for children. The books can be used independently or in concert with its companion book.

As the adult learns the techniques described in a book, they assist the child on their journey through the same topic.

Each book has crossover activities to engage both the adults and children.

In this book, a page with a green ball indicates an opportunity to work with your junior juggling companion.

Not only are you helping your companion prepare to learn juggling, you are sharing experiences in a fun and engaging way.

Introduction

Many years ago I taught myself how to juggle, mostly from sheer boredom at work. Using balled up duct tape I practiced and practiced until I could keep all three balls up in the air continuously. Without the aid of a "how to juggle" book, it took me a long time but the satisfaction of achievement was still there.

Later I taught my family how to juggle and we enjoyed the opportunities to practice together. My son, Andy, really took off and became an accomplished juggler on his own. We started a juggling club in the community where students earned achievement patches. Eventually, we decided to write this book.

Juggling is like a wild violet, plant a seed and watch it take over. Most jugglers not only love to juggle but they love to teach others. That's one of the things I really enjoy about juggling. No matter who you are, no matter what age, regardless of your athletic prowess, you can learn to juggle and be a part of a growing community.

- Mike Murphy

Table of Contents

Why Juggle 9

History of Juggling 12

Making Juggling Balls 17

Warm Up Exercises 21

Juggling Balls........... 23

One Ball 24

Two Balls 28

Three Ball-Hold One........... 32

Three Ball-All Drop 36

Three Ball-Drop One 39

Three Ball Cascade........... 42

Three Ball-One Overhand 47

Ping-Pong........... 50

Juggling Clubs........... 53

One Club........... 56

Two Club Toss........... 59

Two Balls-One Club........... 61

Three Club Cascade 62

Practicing Pointers 66

Juggling Rings 67

Fun Things to Try 72

Table Juggling........... 73

Why Juggle

Low Equipment Cost

Juggling doesn't require professional equipment. You can find things at the dollar store to juggle (glassware not recommended). You can even make your own juggling balls. More on that later in the book.

Improved Hand/Eye Coordination

Juggling creates a strong link between your visual and motor skills.

Challenging and Progressive

The great thing about juggling is that you are always improving your techniques and embracing new challenges. Once you master the basic Three Ball Cascade you can learn Overhand, Ping-Pong, Clawing, and Mills Mess. You'll find yourself juggling different objects and combining tricks into new routines.

Brain Power

There is even some research to suggest that juggling can actually increase brain power. To test that hypothesis, go up to any juggler and ask them a hard question. Just make sure it's about juggling.

No Age Limit

Kids from 8 to 80 can learn to juggle. A co-worker of mine had always wanted to juggle but thought he could never learn. Using the methods in this book he succeeded in one of his lifetime dreams. He now uses that experience as inspiration to overcome other obstacles. "If I can learn to juggle I learn anything".

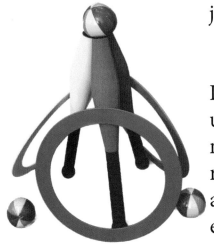

Stress Relieving

If you are feeling down or uninspired, juggle for 15 minutes. Juggling can help relieve stress, depression and anxiety. As with any exercise, juggling can help release endorphins which are feel-good transmitters in your brain. With juggling you forget about the day's stresses and concentrate on your routines and patterns.

Juggling is Portable

You can juggle almost anywhere. We often take juggling balls with us wherever we go in case the opportunity to practice arises. But be aware, juggling can draw crowds of people, especially children.

How to Use this Book

If you follow the methods in this book you will learn to juggle. Juggling is a skill that needs to be learned and practiced. Each exercise in this book builds on the previous exercise, so following the steps in order is important. At the end of each activity, there is a QR code which will take you to a webpage with a video demonstration of the techniques. The images in the book are helpful but often you may need to see the technique demonstrated.

Again, make sure you have mastered each level before moving forward. There are also tips to help you improve your technique.

History of Juggling

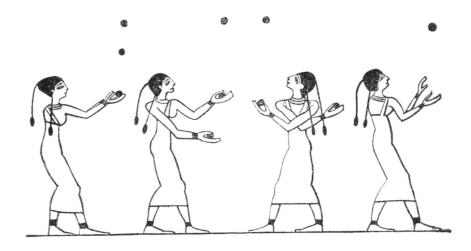

The word juggler comes from the late 14th century Middle English word Jogelen. It means keeping several objects in the air in a continuous motion. As a juggler you will be a member of an ancient brotherhood and sisterhood. Here is a brief history of the major juggling highlights. Read carefully, there will be a quiz (not really).

Archaeologists discovered what is considered the earliest evidence of juggling in the home of an Egyptian prince. The time was between 1194 BCE and 1781 BCE. The wall painting featured several women juggling with three balls, with one of the women juggling with her arms crossed, a great trick.

There are juggling stories of an ancient Chu warrior from China named Xiong Yiliao. Research on Xiong Yiliao dates back to 613-591 BCE. Legend has it that he would juggle either nine balls or seven swords, (research seems to vary) in battle and intimidate

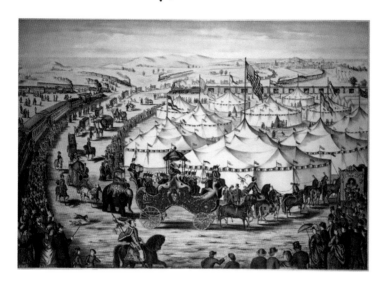

the enemy so much that they turned and ran. I never found juggling intimidating but nine balls is impressive, seven swords more so.

Curiously, ancient Chinese jugglers tended to be warriors. There are references to jugglers throughout Chinese art and literature. Juggling in ancient China was considered an art form and was well respected.

In the medieval period, 5th to 14th century jugglers

were popular because of their whimsy and charm. They were often depicted in artwork of the period.

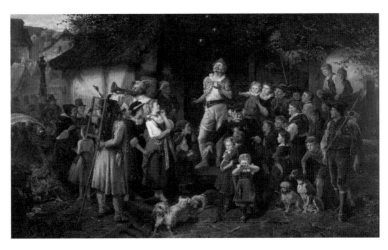

The Juggler-A Village Fair, 1873

In Ireland in the 1500s, jugglers, by law, had to pay a fine to anyone who was hurt from a falling juggling ball or club. After a time, juggling became unfashionable. Jugglers then would only perform in market places and fairs.

In the 1890s, Vaudeville became a celebrated form of entertainment in the United States. Vaudeville would feature 8-10 acts repeated throughout the day. Jugglers were used to fill time between acts. When Vaudeville couldn't compete with the introduction of movies and then television, jugglers were no longer needed.

The Awesome Companion Book of Juggling

Many juggling historians consider Enrico Rastelli, born in Samera, Russia in 1896, one of the greatest jugglers of all time. Coming from a circus family, he reportedly juggled 10 balls, 8 sticks (small clubs) and 8 plates. Probably not all at once.

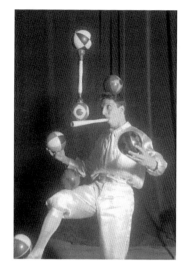

Enrico Rastelli

The International Jugglers Association was founded in 1947 as an organization for jugglers. By then, jugglers were considered professional and legitimate performers and enrollment grew. They currently run a series of workshops and have an annual convention each year.

Since 1971, Madison Area Jugglers Club, in Madison, Wisconsin, hosts Mad Fest in January where you can meet and share techniques with experienced jugglers. The last day of Mad Fest features a juggling extravaganza where professional jugglers show off their skills. It's a great opportunity to meet and learn from other jugglers.

So, as you can see, juggling has had its "ups and downs" with a long and rich history.

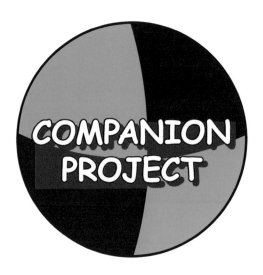

COMPANION PROJECT

Here is an opportunity to work with your companion on a creative project, making juggling balls.

You can purchase quality juggling balls online or at a juggling store (if you can find one) but there is a certain sense of pride and accomplishment in making your own. You can also exercise your creativity by adding stickers and experimenting with different colors.

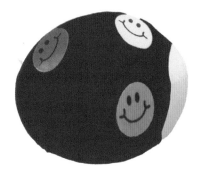

Making Juggling Balls

If you don't want to make an investment in professional juggling balls (at least not yet) here is a fun and easy way to make your own.

Tools and supplies needed

- Scissors
- (3) fold and close sandwich bags
- (6) 12 inch balloons
- 1/2 cup measure of rice, birdseed or sand
- Assorted stickers (optional)
- 1/2 cup measure

First, choose two balloons preferably of different colors.

Cut the top off both balloons. (See figure 1)

Fill a "fold and close" sandwich bag with 1/2 cup of one of the following fillers: birdseed, rice or sand. Rice is a preferred filler. If you use birdseed make sure there are no large seeds that could tear the ball from the inside. Sand works but your juggling balls will be much heavier. (See figure 2)

Take the top of the first balloon and use it to close the bag like a rubber band.

Insert the bag into one of the balloons and pull the balloon over the filled sandwich bag.
(See figure 3)

Take the other balloon and pull it over the first filled balloon, covering the opening. (See figure 4)

Decorate the balls with stickers. You can also cut small holes in the outer balloon revealing the inner balloon color. (See figure 5)

Now, repeat the process two more times to complete your three ball set.

If you're impatient or don't have any balloons you can always use rolled up socks instead.

Watch the complete video on making juggling balls.

https://www.retrorangerpub.com/making-juggling-balls

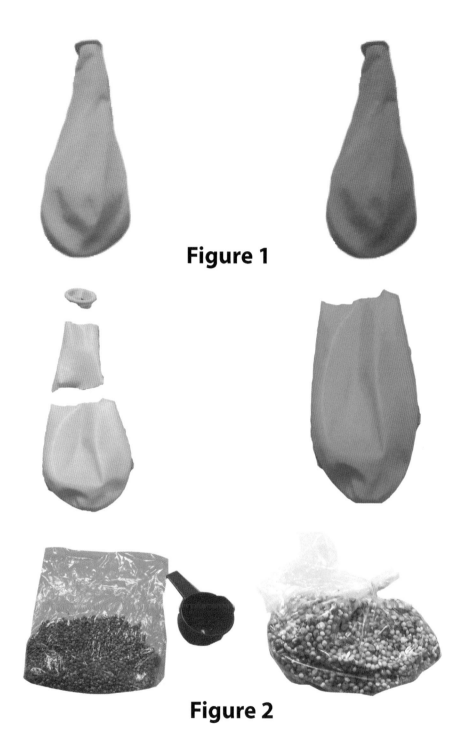

Figure 1

Figure 2

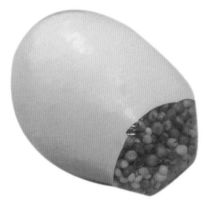

Figure 3

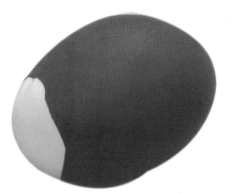

Figure 4

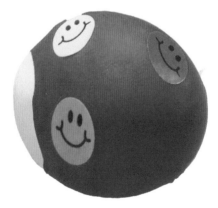

Figure 5

The Awesome Companion Book of Juggling

Warm Up Exercises

Juggling three balls for an extended period of time requires a lot of upper body strength and stamina.

Performing some light upper body exercises can help.

There are many options for upper body strengthening such as resistance bands or light weights. Find one of the many online fitness sites for an exercise routine that works best for you.

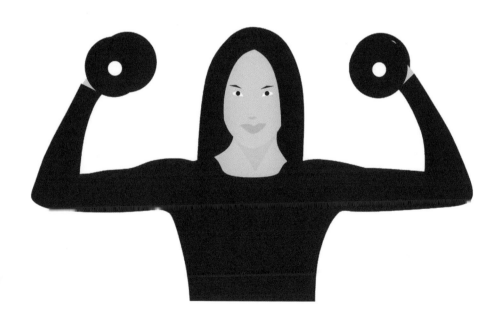

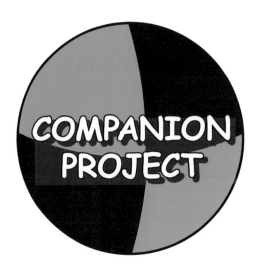

COMPANION PROJECT

Easy and non-stressful warm up exercises are a great opportunity to work with your juggling companion. Since juggling is considered a form of exercise, you should prepare your muscles through a series of warm up activities. It also helps you mentally prepare for each juggling session.

However, we recommend against engaging in any aerobic or weight lifting with a young person. Light stretching alone or with an exercise band is enough to get the blood flowing. Check with your doctor before beginning any type of exercise program.

Juggling Balls

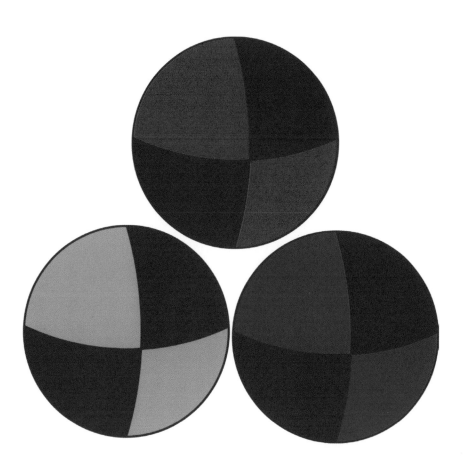

One Ball

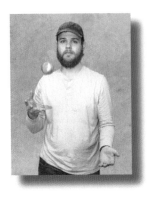

Let's begin your excellent juggling adventure by introducing you to the basics. Mastering these next few exercises will lay the foundation for three ball juggling.

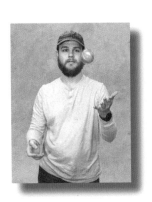

Take one ball and toss it in an arc at eye level height to the other hand and then back again. You are practicing tossing and catching.

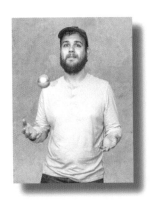

Keep a relaxed stance, arms in toward your body and keep the hands straight out. Try not to move your hands closer together or move your arms up to catch the ball. The goal is to keep a steady, eye level arc.

Once you can consistently toss the ball back and forth in an arc, move on to the next level.

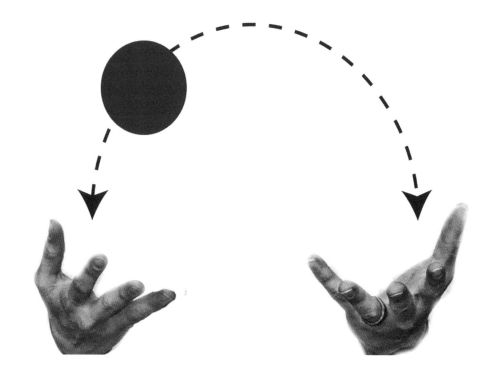

This diagram demonstrates tossing the ball from the right hand to the left hand. Keep your hands open and don't grab the juggling balls. Make sure the ball is arcing back and forth at eye level. Don't reach up to catch the ball, just let it fall into your hands.

Scan the QR Code to see the video.

https://www.retrorangerpub.com/juggling-one-ball-arch

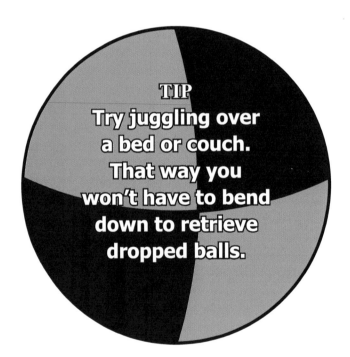

TIP
Try juggling over
a bed or couch.
That way you
won't have to bend
down to retrieve
dropped balls.

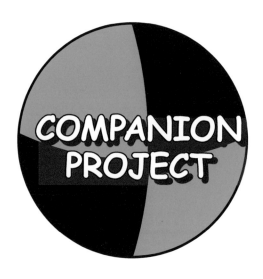

The Awesome Companion Book for Junior Jugglers is filled with fun games that help children develop the skills to move on to beginning juggling. Play next to your companion while they step through each exercise (but don't call it an exercise, that might scare them off).

For example, the first several "games" in the junior juggling book involve either bouncing or rolling a ball against a wall. Sit next to your companion and do the same exercise. Offer positive encouragement, never criticism, and provide assistance when necessary.

There are many opportunities in the junior juggling book for two people to play together. Volunteer to be a companion, even if it means getting on your knees.

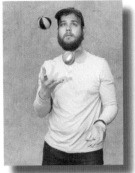

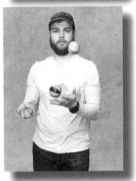

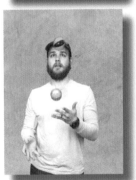

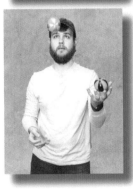

Two Balls

Hold your hands out like you did with the one ball arc, this time with one ball in each hand. Toss the first ball with your dominant hand. When the ball reaches eye level toss the second ball. The goal is to create a crisscross pattern.

If you become frustrated here's a technique you can try. Holding both juggling balls, toss the first ball then toss the second ball. Catch the first ball but let the second ball fall to the ground. Keep practicing until you can finally catch that second ball.

Next, practice keeping the balls moving without dropping. Count your successful volleys and add to that number each time you practice.

The Awesome Companion Book of Juggling

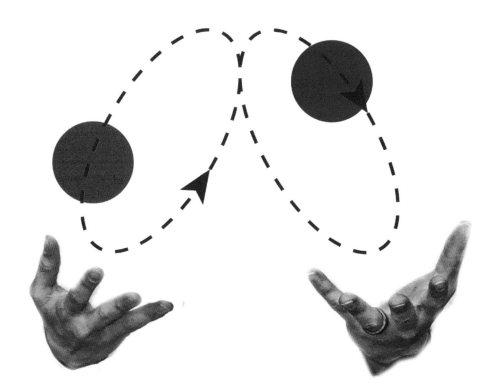

This illustration demonstrates tossing two balls in an arc pattern. Toss the first ball. When it reaches the top of the arc, which should be at eye level, then toss the other ball.

Keep the pattern going. Your goal is to perform consistent repetitions without dropping a ball.

Scan the QR Code to see the video.

https://www.retrorangerpub.com/juggling-two-ball-arch-1

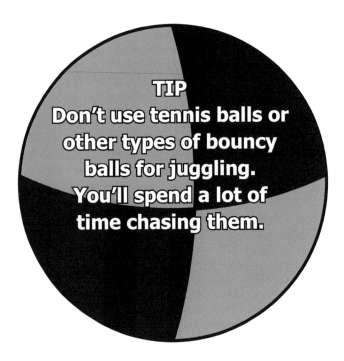

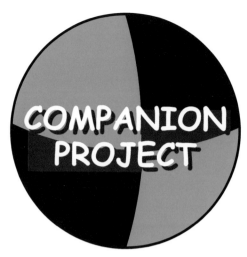

COMPANION PROJECT

Practicing juggling through repetitions is the best way to master the skill. Work with your companion in keeping track of the number of successful throws and catches. Keep a chart that sets reasonable goals. For instance, your chart could be divided into increments of ten such as 10, 20, 30, 40 throws and catches without dropping or losing control of the ball. (See page 75)

Skill	20	30	40
One Ball Arc			
Two Ball Arc			
Three Ball Hold One			

Three Ball-Hold One

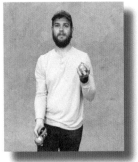

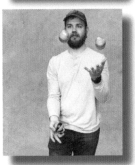

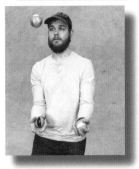

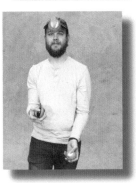

Continue with the two ball crisscross except this time place two balls in one hand and one ball in the other. The purpose of this exercise is to get used to having two balls in one hand while juggling.

With three ball juggling, you begin by having two balls in one hand and one ball in the other. Mastering the Three Ball-Hold One technique is an important step toward three ball juggling.

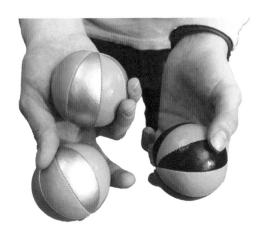

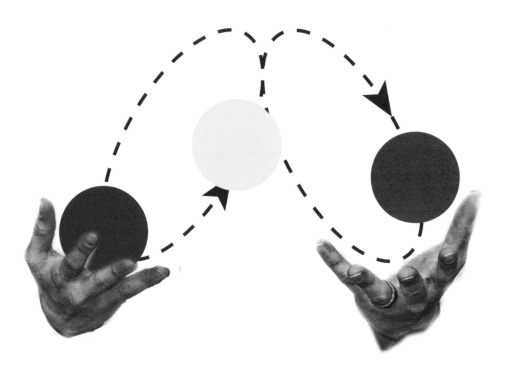

Here is an illustration demonstrating the Three Ball-Hold One technique. The yellow and red ball are tossed in a two ball arc while the blue ball remains in the dominant hand.

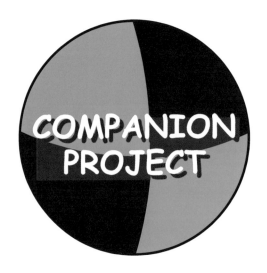

COMPANION PROJECT

If you repeat the same action over and over again you will start to develop muscle memory. Eventually over time the actions become natural, like swimming or riding a bike. You can perform with skill and speed without having to concentrate on what you are doing.

Work with your companion to develop muscle memory for juggling. A simple game of catch, where you keep your palms open when throwing and catching, will train hands not to grab or hold the ball. The ball should fly out of your hands quickly and easily.

The Awesome Companion Book of Juggling

Scan the QR Code to see the video.

https://www.retrorangerpub.com/juggling-three-bal

TIP
Stand relaxed but
straight when juggling.
Beginning jugglers tend to
walk forward as they juggle.
Pretend there is a wall in
front of you that will
stop you from
moving forward.

Three Ball-All Drop

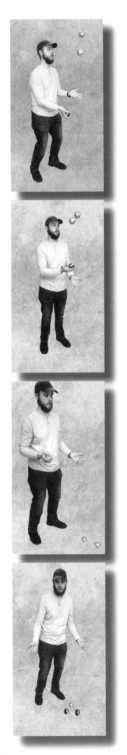

Beginning jugglers often find it difficult to toss the third ball in order to complete a Three Ball Cascade. You have to train your hand to let go of the third ball.

In this exercise you will toss all three balls in a left-right-left pattern or a right-left-right pattern (depending on your dominant hand). Instead of catching the balls, you let the balls drop on the ground.

Done correctly (and if you use non-bouncing balls) the balls should form a loose triangle pattern on the ground.

Scan the QR Code to see the video.

https://www.retrorangerpub.com/three-ball-no-catch

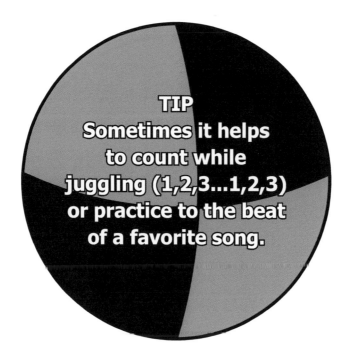

TIP
Sometimes it helps
to count while
juggling (1,2,3...1,2,3)
or practice to the beat
of a favorite song.

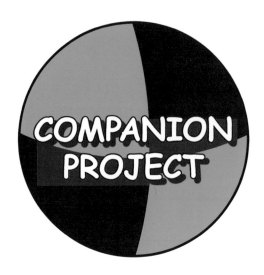

Constant encouragement is important to anyone who is trying something new but especially with young people.

Always be positive and offer words of support when working with a junior juggler. For each successful attempt, praise and urge them on. Even unsuccessful attempts deserve a cheer for the effort.

We found that words of encouragement are great motivators and help provide the incentive to move forward.

Three Ball-Drop One

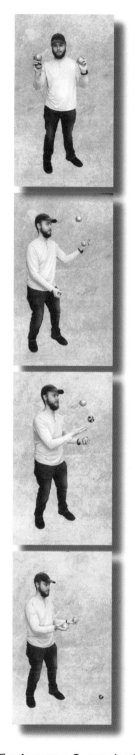

This exercise is similar to the Three Ball-Hold One technique except instead of holding on to the third ball, you toss it.

There is no need to catch the third ball at this stage. Just toss the third ball and let it fall to the ground.

Many people struggle with this exercise. For some reason your hand just doesn't want to let go of that third ball. Of course it has to if you want to advance to Three Ball Cascade.

Just keep practicing the pattern 1-2-toss, 1-2-toss. Catching the third ball comes later.

Scan the QR Code to see the video.

https://www.retrorangerpub.com/three-ball-no-catch

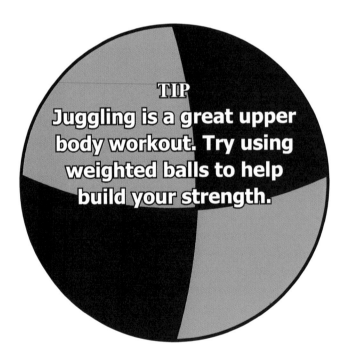

TIP
Juggling is a great upper body workout. Try using weighted balls to help build your strength.

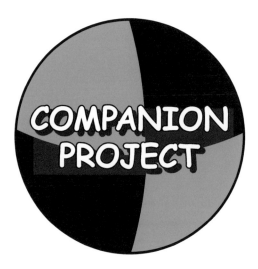

COMPANION PROJECT

Here's a great game you can play with your companion. Stand side by side both facing forward. With your outside hands toss a ball to each other. Maintain a good arc and rhythm. At some point switch sides to practice with the other hand. Remember, cup the ball don't grab it. For an extra challenge, try adding a second ball.

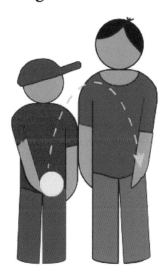

Three Ball Cascade

When most people think of juggling they picture a person tossing and catching three balls in the air. All the exercises up to this point were designed to prepare you for this level.

Naturally, the next step is to toss the third ball back into the pattern and keep all three balls constantly moving. This is known as a Three Ball Cascade. In Three Ball Cascade each ball must follow the same pattern and rhythm as the previous ball and the pattern must be continuous.

Keep track of the number of times you can maintain the cascade without dropping a ball. Try to build on that number each time you practice. The thrill of accomplishment will come when you are able to keep tossing and catching the balls consistently like a true juggler.

A great way to understand the pattern and technique of three ball juggling is to go to Andy's video via the QR code or the URL provided on page 45. Watch it several times, if necessary, to become familiar with the routine.

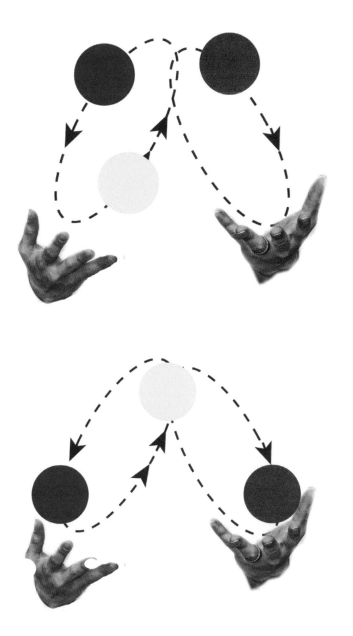

These illustrations demonstrate the flow and direction of the Three Ball Cascade

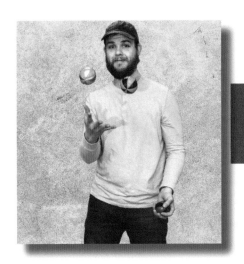

KEEP

ON

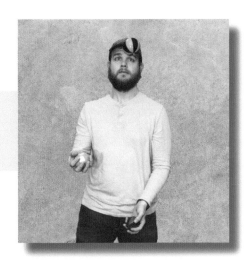

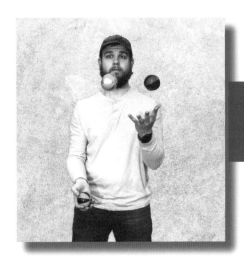

JUGGLING

The Awesome Companion Book of Juggling

Scan the QR Code to see the video.

https://www.retrorangerpub.com/three-ball-cascade

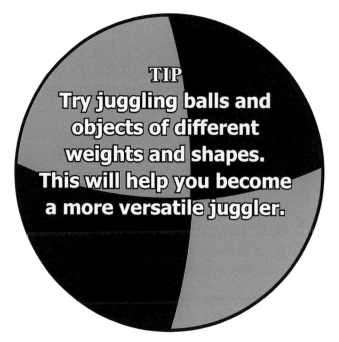

TIP
Try juggling balls and
objects of different
weights and shapes.
This will help you become
a more versatile juggler.

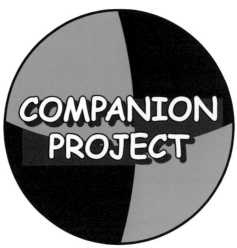

In <u>The Awesome Companion Book for Junior Jugglers</u> there are levels, represented by animals, to recognize achievement goals.

Help your companion earn those levels and celebrate those accomplishments. Here are the levels in order.

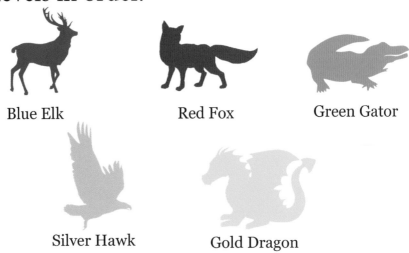

Blue Elk   Red Fox   Green Gator

Silver Hawk   Gold Dragon

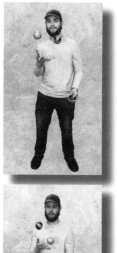

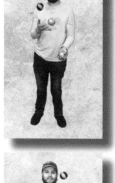

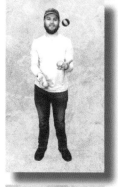

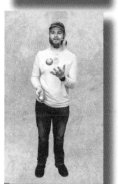

Three Ball-One Overhand

After you have established a good rhythm with the Three Ball Cascade, begin randomly tossing one ball overhand instead of underhand.

Keep the rhythm going and try another overhand toss using your dominant hand. Later practice tossing overhand with your non-dominant hand.

If you find this difficult, try one, two, three, over, catch, stop. Then start again, one, two, three, over, catch, stop to get used to tossing the ball overhand.

With practice, you can add an overhand toss into your juggling routine.

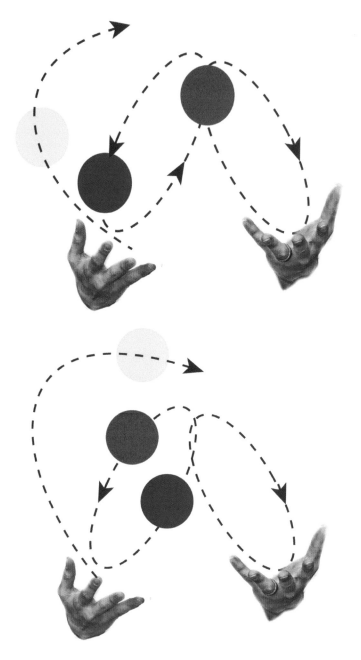

The yellow ball is tossed overhand instead of underhand.

The Awesome Companion Book of Juggling

Scan the QR Code to see the video.

**https://www.retrorangerpub.com/
juggling-three-ball-one-overhand**

TIP
**It's great to juggle
with a friend. Find
someone who can juggle
or would like to learn to
juggle using this book.
You can challenge and
encourage each other.**

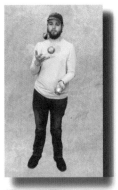

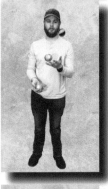

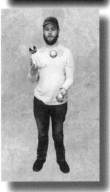

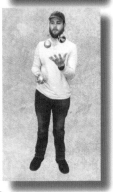

Ping-Pong

Now that you've practiced the Three Ball-One Overhand exercise, you can move on to Ping-Pong. Ping-Pong is like playing hot potato with a single specific ball in your cascade.

With Ping-Pong, instead of tossing random balls in an overhand pattern, you choose just one ball. It's like a Ping-Pong ball bouncing back and forth between players but in this case the Ping-Pong ball is your juggling ball and your hands are the paddles.

Use your most colorful or distinct juggling ball as your Ping-Pong candidate so it is easy for you, and your audience to see the Ping-Pong effect.

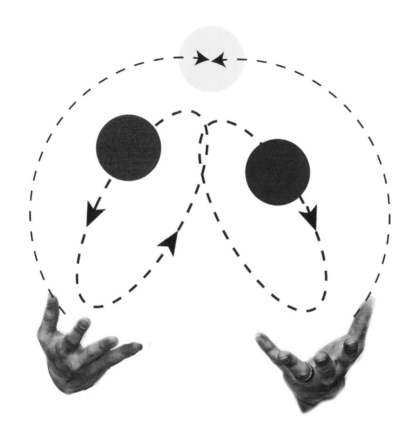

Ping-Pong

This pattern is very similar to the Three Ball-One Overhand pattern except in this case you toss the same ball back and forth overhand like a Ping-Pong ball between paddles. See how the same yellow ball is passed overhand back and forth.

Scan the QR Code to see the video.

https://www.retrorangerpub.com/juggling-ping-pong

TIP
See if there is a juggling club in your area. If not, start one. Working with others helps build confidence and sharpens your skill set.

Juggling Clubs

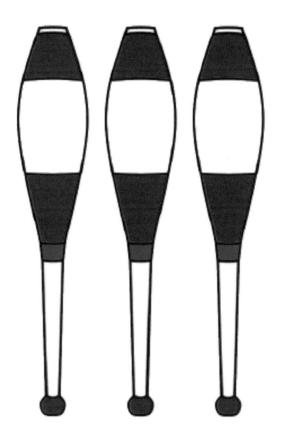

Clubs

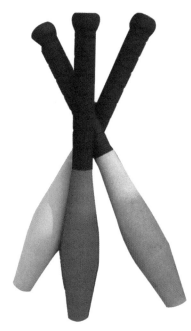

Working with clubs is the next step in your juggling journey. Juggling clubs are generally shaped like a bowling pin with a long neck handle that widens at the end. They are also available in various lengths, widths and styles.

The best clubs are well balanced toward the center making juggling much easier. You can purchase clubs from stores that sell professional juggling equipment. For beginners I would recommend clubs with a soft covering on the handle to avoid painful hands. I found a great, inexpensive set online covered in high density foam. Do some research for clubs that best meet your comfort level.

Club juggling is visually exciting and fascinating to watch. You apply the same skills you learned from the Three Ball Cascade except, this time, you are spinning clubs instead of tossing balls.

We recommend that you practice in a large, clear area with a fairly high ceiling. Outside is great, if it's not windy. Wind makes it much more difficult to control the clubs.

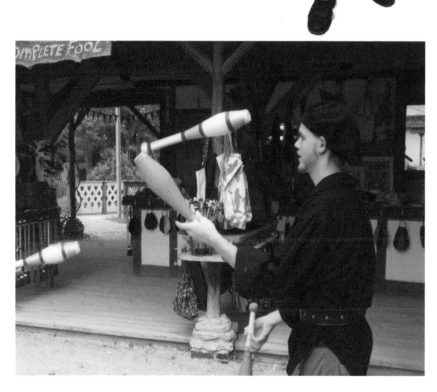

One Club

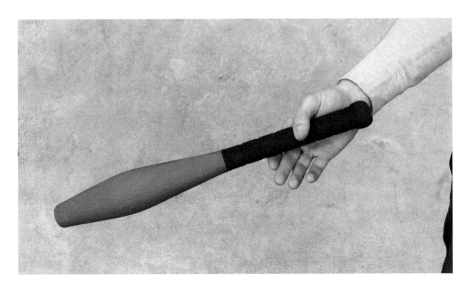

To begin club juggling, start with one club. Hold the club about a third of the way up the handle. Don't grip the club tightly like someone is going to steal it but instead hold the club somewhat loose.

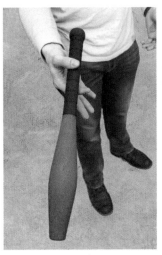

Balance the club with your thumb on top and the club handle resting on your forefinger and middle finger.

Toss the club gently one rotation, catching the handle about a third of the way up. You'll have less control of the club if you catch it at the knob end.

The Awesome Companion Book of Juggling

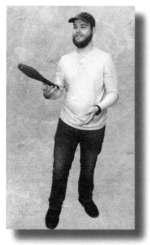

When practicing, stand up straight and keep your hand down near your waist. Toss the club one revolution to eye level height and let the club fall back into your hand. It will take practice to develop the muscle memory to toss the club with just the right amount of force.

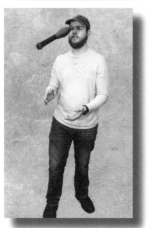

When you are comfortable tossing with each hand independently, you can practice tossing continuously back and forth between hands.

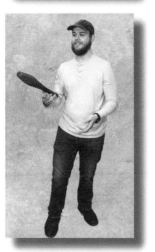

Practice tossing the club from your dominant hand to your non-dominant hand one rotation per toss. After several repetitions, begin tossing from your non-dominant to your dominant hand.

Scan the QR Code to see the video.

https://www.retrorangerpub.com/juggling-one-club

TIP
Learning to juggle clubs can get a little frustrating. Set aside a time to practice and set a goal each day. You are trying to develop muscle memory so tossing and catching the club becomes second nature.

Two Club Toss

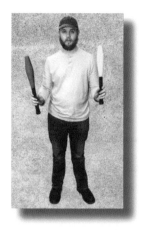

Toss two clubs back and forth between your hands similar to the two ball arc. Spin the clubs one revolution each time you toss them, catching the handle. It is common to toss the clubs high but work to keep the clubs at eye level.

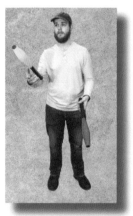

Begin with a simple pattern of up, up, catch, catch, then start again. This will help you build muscle memory and maintain a consistent spin and height for the clubs.

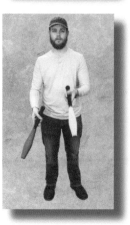

Resist the tendency to walk forward while juggling two clubs. However, intentional walking while juggling is a skill you can develop later.

Scan the QR Code to see the video.

https://www.retrorangerpub.com/juggling-two-club

TIP
Try to keep the speed of your spins consistent. Tossing one club faster than the other makes it difficult to maintain a steady uniform pattern.

Two Balls-One Club

Before you begin tossing three clubs, here is an intermediate step that some people find helpful.

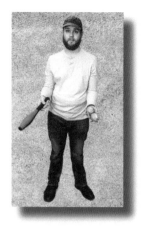

Begin by holding two balls in your dominant hand and the club in the other hand. Start the cascade as you would with three balls. The pattern will be ball-club-ball.

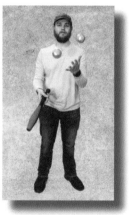

This is not an essential exercise. Some people want to jump right into three club juggling and that's fine. But if you find yourself struggling try this transitional step.

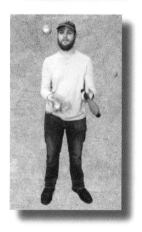

Three Club Cascade

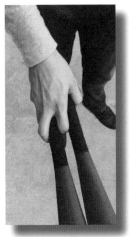

Mastering club juggling takes a lot of practice but it is worth it. It's an incredible feeling when you can keep the cascade going with clubs but it will challenge your upper body strength.

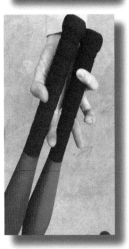

Hold two clubs in your dominant hand, one on top of the other, using your index finger as a spacer. Hold the third club in the other hand.

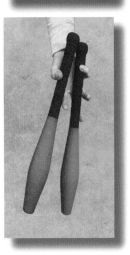

Begin by tossing the top club from your dominant hand followed by the club from the other hand.

Continue with the cascade, tossing each club one revolution into the air at eye level.

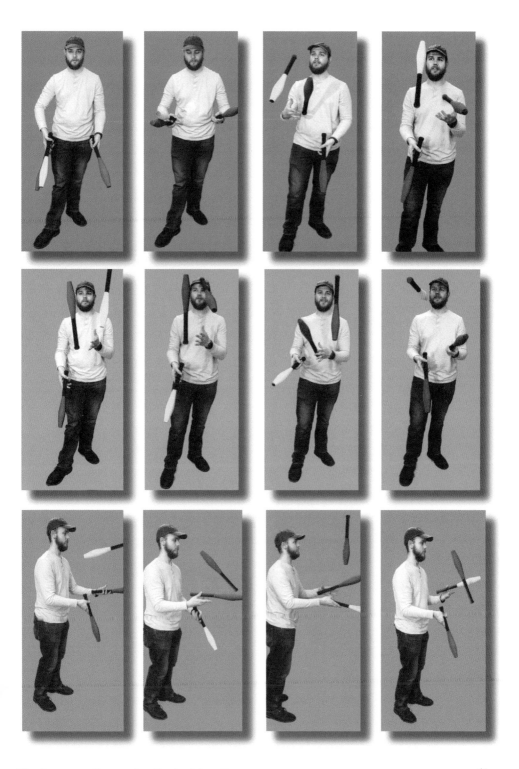

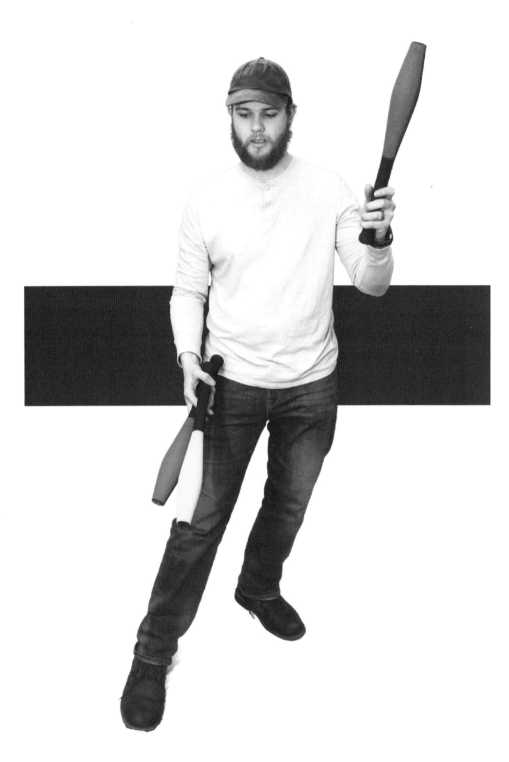

The Awesome Companion Book of Juggling

Scan the QR Code to see the video.

https://www.retrorangerpub.com/juggling-three-club-cascade

TIP
To avoid hurt hands and fingers when juggling clubs, purchase beginner foam covered clubs online. Also, always catch the clubs in the middle of the handle. This will help prevent pinched fingers.

Practicing Pointers

Walking Forward

You may have a tendency to move forward when you first practice club juggling. Pretty soon you've walked around the block trying to keep up with the clubs. Keep your feet firmly on the ground and toss the clubs straight up and not forward.

Juggling Too Fast

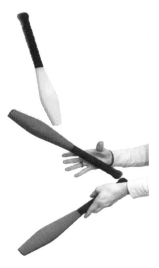

Don't rush through the juggling pattern. Start at a slower pace until you can consistently maintain the cascade for 30 seconds or more without dropping a club. Keep practicing the cascade for 40 seconds, 50 seconds, one minute and so on.

Take a Break

Take a break long before you get frustrated or tired. Let your muscles rest awhile before juggling again. . A good rule of thumb is to practice for 20 minutes, take a break for 5 minutes, and practice again for 20 minutes. Often you'll find you can juggle better after a break.

The Awesome Companion Book of Juggling

Juggling Rings

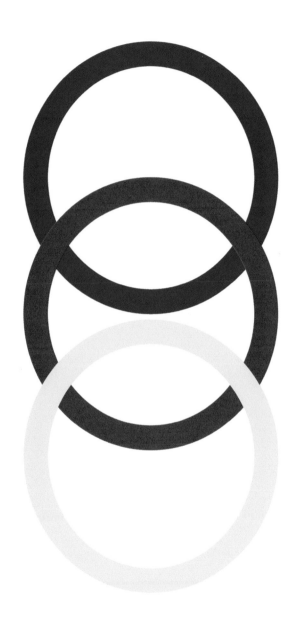

Rings

Juggling rings is a lot of fun. Like clubs, rings are a very visual form of juggling. Brightly colored rings flying in the air is a great show and, in our opinion, easier to juggle than clubs.

Just like juggling balls and clubs, begin by practicing with one ring and one hand. It's important to spin the ring while you are tossing it in the air. Putting a good spin on the ring provides more control when catching. You will have to experiment with the speed of the spin so the ring stays straight in the air without wobbling.

The next step is to toss the ring from one hand to the other while maintaining the spin. Toss the ring at eye level or slightly above.

The Awesome Companion Book of Juggling

Now try working with two rings tossing them back and forth between your hands. Keep the same rhythm as with ball and club juggling.

When you are confident with your ability to toss and catch the two rings consistently, introduce the third ring into the cascade.

This picture demonstrates the best way to hold two rings for juggling.

We recommend not practicing outside on a windy day. It is very hard to control your rings under those conditions.

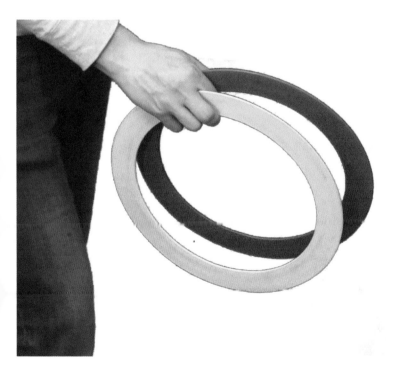

One Ring

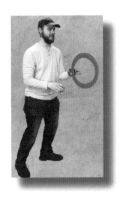 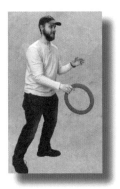 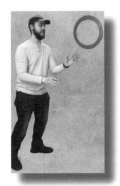 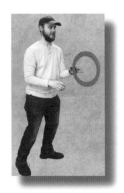

Two Rings

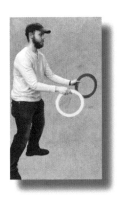 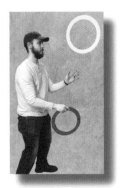 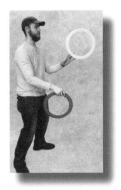 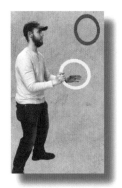

Three Rings

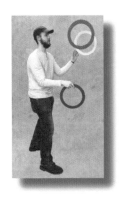 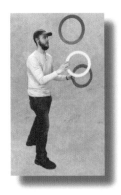 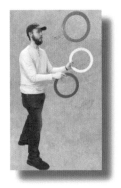 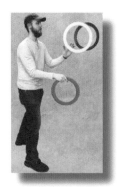

The Awesome Companion Book of Juggling

Scan the QR Code to see the video.

https://www.retrorangerpub.com/juggling-one-ring

TIP
You can purchase tossing rings at most department stores but the best option is to purchase a professional set of rings that are specifically balanced for juggling.

Fun Things to Try

Try walking forward then backward while you are juggling. Just make sure the area is clear ahead and behind.

Joggling is a sport where contestants juggle while jogging. Some competitors joggle a mile on a track.

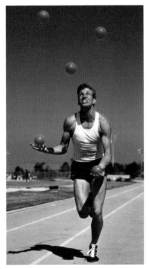
Joggling

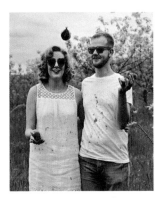
Side by Side
Emilie and Andy

Try side by side. Perform a Three Ball Cascade shoulder to shoulder with another juggler using one set of juggling balls.

Three ball flash. Toss all three balls up in the air with one hand and then catch the balls to begin your cascade.

Carry juggling balls with you at all times. You can even get (or make) a set of small juggling balls. Cylindrical pencil cases make great juggling ball cases. Attach it to your belt with a carabiner.

The Awesome Companion Book of Juggling

Table Juggling

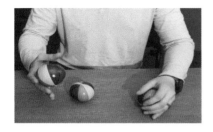 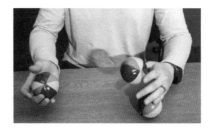

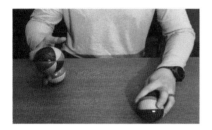 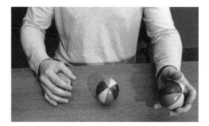

Scan the QR Code to see the video.

https://www.retrorangerpub.com/juggling-table-top-juggling

So where do you go from here? That is the beauty of juggling. There is no limit to the possibilities you can explore. The International Juggling Association is a great resource for juggling programs, activities, tips and tutorials. You can always find jugglers demonstrating their skills on YouTube or other social media sites.

Check out these "Razzle Dazzle" videos of fun juggling techniques.

Scan the QR Code to see the video.

https://www.retrorangerpub.com/juggling-razzle-dazzle-one

https://www.retrorangerpub.com/juggling-razzle-dazzle-two

	20	30	40
One Ball Arc			
Two Ball Arc			
Two Balls Hold One			
Three Balls All Drop			
Three Balls Drop One			
Three Ball Cascade			
Three Balls One Overhand			
Ping Pong			
One Club			
Two Clubs			
Three Club Cascade			
Rings			

About the Authors

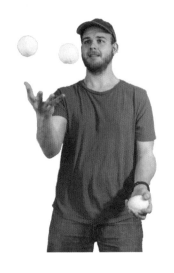

Andy Murphy is an accomplished juggler and musician. He has been juggling for more than 14 years and is a proud member of the International Juggling Association. Andy is the co-founder of the BCR Juggling Club in Kenosha, Wisconsin. Andy resides in Wisconsin with his wife, Emilie, and their daughter, Dolly.

Mike Murphy is also a 14 year veteran of juggling and co-founder of the BCR Juggling Club. Mike lives in Kenosha, Wisconsin with his wife, Gail. Oh, and he's Andy's father.

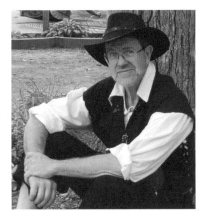

Mike at the Bristol Renaissance Fair. A great place to observe jugglers.

Acknowledgements

History of Juggling

https://en.wikipedia.org/wiki/History_of_juggling

A Brief History of Juggling

http://www.juggling.org/books/artists/history.html

From "Juggling, the Art and its Artists", by Karl-Heinz Ziethen and Andrew Allen, Berlin 1985

Research in Juggling History

By Professor Arthur Lewbel

https://www2.bc.edu/arthur-lewbel/jugweb/history-1.html

https://commons.wikimedia.org/wiki/File:Fritz_Beinke_-_The_juggler-_a_village_fair_-_Google_Art_Project.jpg

Juggling -Its History and Greatest Performers by Francisco Alvarez

http://www.juggling.org/books/alvarez/part1.html

How Juggling Works by Jonathan Strickland

https://entertainment.howstuffworks.com/juggling11.htm

Joggling at en.wikipediaen.wikipedia, Public Domain, https://commons.wikimedia.org/w/index.php?curid=3851125

Original uploader was RadioKirk (image)

Images on pages 12, 13, 14, 15, 72 are in public domain

Special Acknowledgments

Sean Murphy, image on page 6.

Emilie Murphy, Side by Side, image on page 72.

Original music composed and performed by Andy Murphy.

Find other
Awesome Companion Books
and the
Hidden Hollow Tales series of
children's books at
retrorangerpub.com

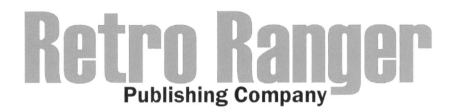

Retro Ranger
Publishing Company

Printed in Great Britain
by Amazon

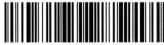